Natural Recipes
to cure:
The Asthma, Asthma Bronchial, Bronchitis, Rhinitis-Sinusitis

Health & Wellness

Natural Recipes
to cure:
The Asthma, Asthma Bronchial, Bronchitis, Rhinitis-Sinusitis

By Silvia Alvarez

May 2020

First Edition May 2020
ISBN KDP No. 9798648303881
Edited by Silvia Alvarez
Copyright © 2020. Silvia Alvarez.
Printed in Perú
No part of this work can be reproduced by any means without the Autor´s permission. The ink we use is clorine free and the inner paper type is acid free. Both products are supplied by a supplier certified by the Forest Stewarchip (FSC Forest Stewarchip)
The paper is made with 30% recicled waste material.

INDEX

Bibliography.
INTRODUCTION
CHAPTER 1
ASTHMA CAN BE CURED?
2.- Recipe No. 2. GINGER:
4.- Recipe No. 4. EUCALYPTUS:
6.- Recipe No. 6. LEMON, ORANGE, CARROT:
CHAPTER 2
NATURAL RECIPES FOR ASTHMATIC COUGH:
4. LEMON JUICE.
7. TURMERIC.
Recipe to cure Asthma forever:
CHAPTER 3
Recipe Preparation for Bronchitis:
3. RECIPE OF GARLIC MILK (CURES ASTHMA)
Preparation Green Mango Recipe:
CHAPTER 4
RECOMMENDATIONS TO COMBAT RHINITIS - SINUSITIS

Bibliography

Querys:

- ✓ Dr. Alonso Vega.
- ✓ National Directorate of Medicines: Health Education Program that addresses issues related to the rational use and consumption of medicines.
- ✓ Tips Dr Sebastian Malek, Dr Mario Solórzano.

Photos: PxFuel, The Stocks.

Written by Silvia A. Alvarez M.

INTRODUCTION

Natural products have a common goal of preventing and treating diseases, this type of medicine is a mixture of all those healing skills that have been part of the cultural heritage of each nation. Its use dates back to ancient times, when man sought remedy for his ills in nature. In this book we present the herbs that are considered the most used, we also indicate precisely why and how the mentioned herbs are prepared, the photos facilitate the understanding of each recipe.

Here we gather some recipes that are used to cure from the flu to asthma, which is the central disease that we will be treating in this book.

The ancient inhabitants of the earth, our ancestors, knew how to use these natural recipes. Healing with plants is as old as people themselves. Consequently, we now know that with herbs we can heal ourselves.

This book was written with the commitment to offer the testimony of healing that can be obtained with the constant use of these recipes, for which I invite you to read and consult it, in the hope that it may be useful in the complete healing of everyone. so need it.

CHAPTER 1

WHAT IS ASTHMA :

Asthma is a condition in which the airways narrow and swell, causing more mucus. This could make it difficult to breathe and cause coughing, wheezing, and shortness of breath.

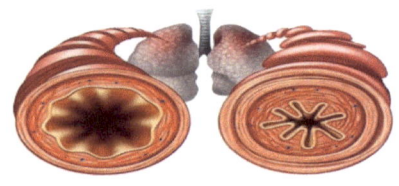

TRIGGERS OF ASTHMA:

Substances found in the air, such as pollen, dust mites, mold spores, pet dander, or cockroach residue particles, physical activity (**Asthma** caused by exercise) Cold air. Air pollutants and irritants, such as smoke.

RECOMMENDATIONS FOR CONTROLLING ASTHMA:

1) Do respiratory exercises daily.

2) Play sports with caution.

3) Do not smoke, do not visit environments with smoke.

4) When you travel keep asthma under control.

5) Take your medication every day, even if you don't have symptoms.

6) Never abandon treatment on your own.

7) Always consult your doctor before taking new drugs.

8) Learn how to use your inhaler well.

9) Learn to recognize and act in the face of crises.

10) You exercise regularly, it will help you strengthen your breathing.

ASTHMA CAN BE CURED?

The **Asthma** is a chronic disease and does not have una definitive cure according to doctors. The treatment provided by doctors allows, in most cases, to be controlled and lead a normal life. The Natural Remedies can help heal definitely this condition, but we must be constant until we see the results we expect. Below I give you a series of recipes with natural ingredients, which we usually have at home, they are very easy to prepare, take note:

NATURAL RECIPES TO HEAL ASTHMA

1.- Recipe No. 1. ONION AND LEMON:

Ingredients:

- 02 Onions
- 02 tablespoons of honey
- 02 Lemon juice.

Preparation:

Cook 2 sliced onions in a skillet for 2 minutes. Add liter of water, let the water reduce to 1/3, add the juice of the 2 lemons, let stand, add 02 tablespoons of honey, strain, place it in a jar. Take 2 tablespoons 3 times a day.

2.- Recipe No. 2. GINGER:

Ingredients:

01 Ginger Root

Preparation:

Place a cup of water in a small saucepan, and add 1/2 ginger root chopped into pieces, once weed, take in the form of tea, fasting and at night, minimum for three months.

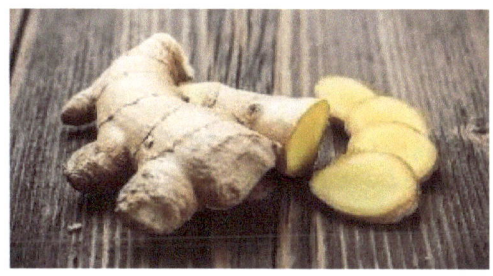

3.- Recipe No. 3. TURMERIC:

Ingredients:

01 Turmeric powder

Preparation:

Place on the fire, in a small pot, a cup of water, and add a teaspoon of turmeric, take as a tea, twice a day: on an empty stomach and at night.

4.- Recipe No. 4. EUCALYPTUS:

Ingredients:

    01 Eucalyptus branches

Preparation:

In a saucepan, add a cup of water, and several eucalyptus leaves, take on an empty stomach and at night.

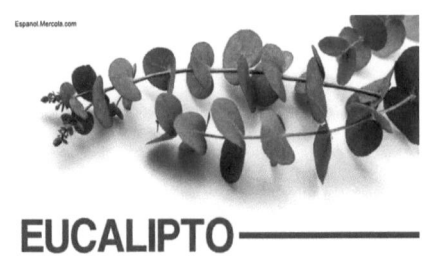

5.- Recipe No. 5. HONEY, LEMON AND GINGER:

Ingredients:

    01 Cup of Honey
    02 Lemons (Lemon Juice)
    01 Ginger Root (small)

Preparation:

Place in the blender, then place in a glass bottle keep inside the fridge (every day take out in a small container (3 shots) what you are going to take, this so that you do not take it cold from the fridge, take it three times a day.

6.- Recipe No. 6. LEMON, ORANGE, CARROT:

Ingredients:

    1/2 lemon (juice)
    03 carrots
    01 Orange
    01 Glass of Water

Preparation:

Put in the blender the orange juice, the lemon juice, chop the carrots into small pieces, along with the glass of water. Then take 3 times a day.

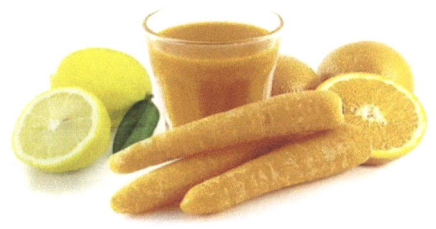

7.- Recipe No. 7. MUSTARD OIL WITH CAMPHOR:

Ingredients:

    Mustard Oil
    Camphor

Preparation:

Put in a container a tablespoon of Mustard Oil, add camphor and massage the chest and back, this will help the person to breathe better.

CHAPTER 2

BRONCHIAL ASTHMA

Bronchial Asthma: It is a lung disease, caused by inflammation and narrowing of the mucous membranes of the bronchi, preventing the correct entry and exit of air from the lungs.

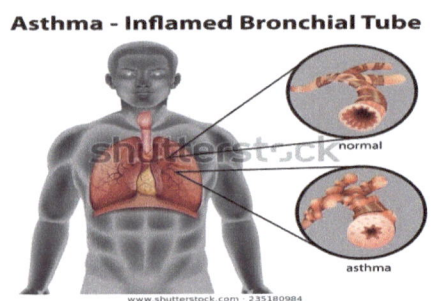

Below we present several Recipes with Natural products that effectively combat it with constant performance:

RECIPE No. 1:

Ingredients:

    02 Onions (Purple preferably)
    07 Lemons
    04 Garlic
    1/2 ginger root
    01 cup of honey

Preparation:

Place everything in the blender without the honey, then strain, add it in a glass container and add the honey, take 3 times a day for 20 continuous days, stop for 10 days, resume again for 20 more days and rest for 10 days, repeat this treatment until the asthma disappears completely, many patients have completely healed from asthma, there are testimonies that certify it. My son started drinking this treatment 20 days ago, and the episodes of bronchial asthma have decreased, with this expectation, she will repeat it for at least 4 months, trusting that it will completely heal.

NATURAL RECIPES FOR ASTHMATIC COUGH:

1. GINGER OR KION: Ginger tea is a natural alternative to relieve asthma, as it has broncho-dilating properties that will help you breathe better. This effect inhibits an enzyme that causes the muscles in the airways to contract, while activating another enzyme that relaxes the airways.

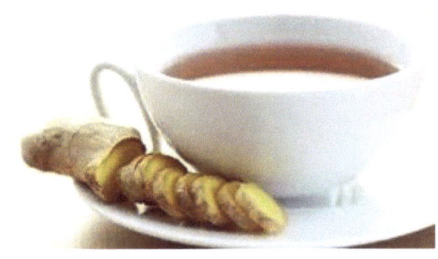

2. ONION: Thanks to the fact that it has a flavonoid called quercetin, the onion helps to relax the bronchi and decrease the constriction of the airways. Among its compounds, there is also thiosulphinates, which is known for its anti-asthmatic properties.

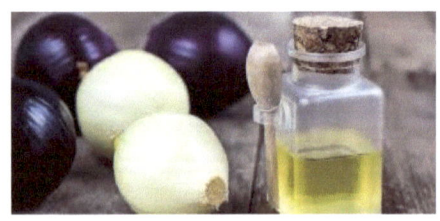

3. GARLIC. Previously, garlic was used as a natural medicine thanks to its anti-inflammatory properties. In fact, garlic extract significantly reduces inflammation of the airways.

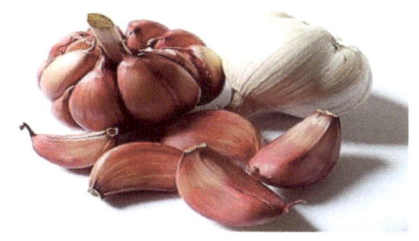

4. LEMON JUICE. It helps prevent mucus from accumulating in the bronchi, improving breathing and cleaning the respiratory system of bacteria and germs that hinder the passage of the air.

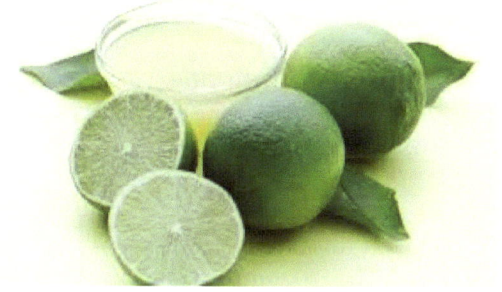

5. HONEY. It is a natural expectorant and anti-inflammatory that helps eliminate phlegm. Is Useful for removing mucus that accumulates in the airways and blocks the flow of air that It could trigger or exacerbate an asthma attack.

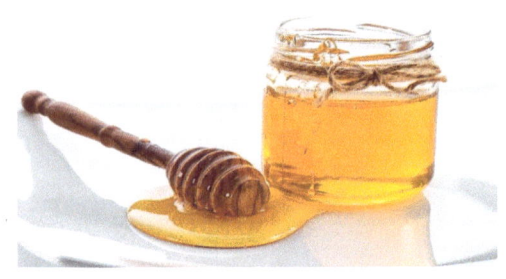

6. GINKGO BILOBA. The leaf inhibits a substance found in the lungs and causes inflammation of the airways. It acts as a broncho dilator and reduces the inflammation, so it is recommended to take twice a day an infusion of Ginkgo biloba.

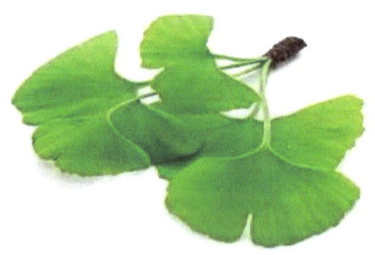

7. TURMERIC. It is a spice with anti-inflammatory and expectorant properties, which helps to naturally control asthma. Turmeric has a protective action on the respiratory system.

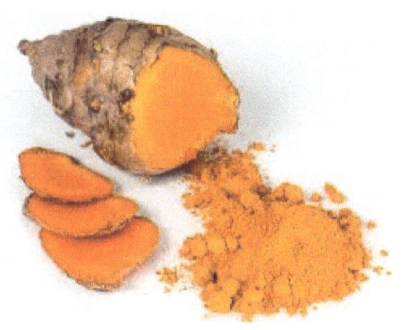

8. **GREEN TEA.** It is a natural source of theophylline, which is a substance with action rough dilator that is part of many drugs used to treat asthma. It relaxes the muscles that support the bronchial tubes, and is used to prevent and treatpuffing, shortness of breath, and shortness of breath.

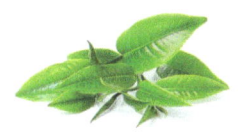

Recipe to cure Asthma forever:

1.- Radish, carrot, onion, lemon and honey recipe:

Ingredients:

- 1 onion
- 3 radishes
- 1 lemon
- 1 carrot
- 2 tablespoons of honey

Preparation:

We remove the shell and the corner of the onion, we make equal to the radish we remove only the corners, we leave the shell, we grate the carrot with the knife to remove the shell, we chop the lemon in 2, we grate the ingredients with a grater on the smaller side, and place everything in a medium-sized pot, place it on the stove in a bain-marie, cover it, let it boil for 30 minutes, once this time has passed, with a cheesecloth, place the ingredients and strain. to squeeze all the juice that the ingredients released on the fire, then we add the lemon juice, add the honey, and place in a glass container.

It is taken 3 times a day, this recipe can be repeated as long as necessary, until the symptoms of asthma completely disappear.

This recipe is effective in eliminating asthma permanently.

Recipe with peppermint and white cane:

Ingredients:

- 1/2 liter of white cane
- 2 bunches of peppermint

Preparation: In a glass bottle of 1 liter, place the half liter of white cane, add the bunch of peppermint there, place it in an outdoor place for 3 days without uncovering. After these three days, start taking two tablespoons on an empty stomach. Take for 20 days, rest 10 days, do this for at least 3 months.

CHAPTER 3

BRONCHITIS

The **bronchitis** is inflammation of the bronchial tubes, the airways that carry oxygen to the lungs This causes a cough that frequently has mucus. It also causes shortness of breath, gasping, and chest pressure. There are two types of **bronchitis**: acute and chronic.

BRONCHIAL ASTHMA:

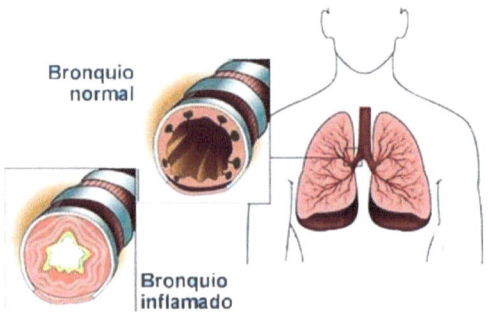

Respiratory system disease characterized by labored and labored breathing, coughing, choking sensation, and wheezing in the chest.

Below we give you several recipes to combat bronchitis and asthma generated by it.

1. RECIPE TO CURE BRONCHITIS:

Ingredients:

- 1/2 cup of milk
- 01 Spoonful of Honey
- 01 tablespoon of butter
- 01 Egg Yolk
- 1/4 tablespoon of baking soda

Recipe Preparation for Bronchitis:

Put the milk to a boil in a small saucepan, remove from the heat, then add the honey, butter, mix well, add the egg yolk and baking soda. Take 5 minutes before sleeping.

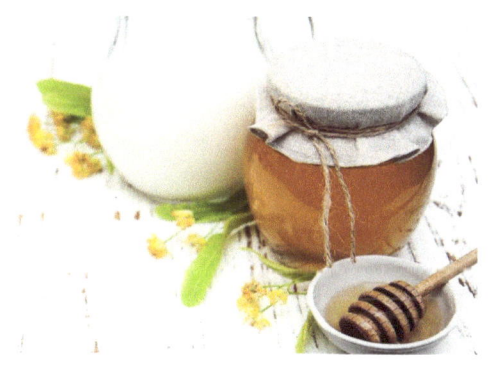

2. JUICE TO FIGHT ASTHMA:

Ingredients:

    03 Kiwi without shell
    01 Apple
    01 large garlic clove
    01 Glass of Water
    01 tablespoon ground flaxseed

Preparation:

Everything is liquefied. It should be taken three (03) times a day, when you do not have asthma. This recipe strengthens the lungs.

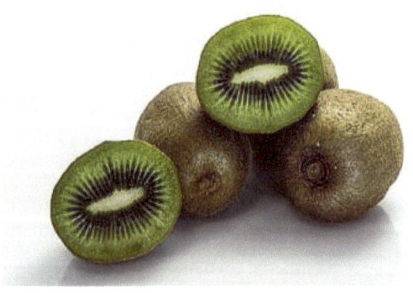

3. RECIPE OF GARLIC MILK (CURES ASTHMA)

Ingredients:

    10 Garlic Cloves
    1/2 liter of milk
    2 or 3 tablespoons of sugar

Preparation:

Boil the milk until the mixture is halved together with the garlic, strain and add the sugar. Take warm 3 times a day.

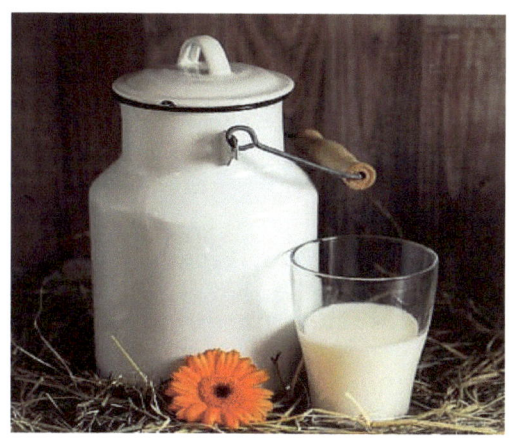

4. RECIPE OF THE THREE (3) GREEN HANDLES:

Ingredients:

    03 Green Mangoes
    1/2 tablespoon of sweet cloves and cinnamon
    2 tablespoons of honey

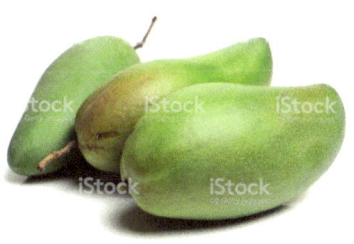

Preparation Green Mango Recipe:

In a medium saucepan, place the green mangoes, add sweet cloves and Cinnamon, place water in the pot that covers the handles, bring to a boil and cover until the water reduces by half, once the water is reduced, put out the fire, Wait for it to cool, remove the seeds from the mangoes and the sweet cloves, and blend. Reserve in a glass container.

Taking 3 times a day, and repeating for a minimum of three months, evaluates the improvements in asthma attacks, and determines whether to continue it for two or three more months, according to the progress you have made.

CHAPTER 4
RHINITIS-SINUSITIS:

The symptoms of sinusitis and of the rhinitisthey are very similar. The rhinitis is an inflammation of the mucous membranes of the nose, while the sinusitis includes inflammation of the sinuses and nasal passages, which It produces sneezing, itching, obstruction, runny nose, and sometimes a lack of smell. These symptoms generally appear for more than 3 consecutive days, it is generally caused by viruses, allergies or pathogens. A fever may also occur, in this case, We must go to the doctor because it can represent an infection that requires taking antibiotics.

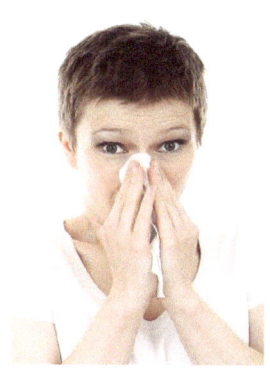

1) RECIPE TO CURE RHINITIS-SINUSITIS:

Ingredients:

- ✓ Sea salt
- ✓ 1 Dropper.
- ✓ 100 ml boiled water
- ✓ 100 ml filtered water

Preparation:

Nasal lavage is done.

Place 1/2 teaspoon of sea salt in 100 ml of boiled water, then add 1/2 cup of filtered water, with this mixture of waters 3 drops are placed in each nostril three times a day. This loosens the mucus and it is easier for you to expel it, that way they disappear accumulated mucus from sinusitis or rhinitis.

RECOMMENDATIONS TO COMBAT RHINITIS - SINUSITIS

a) To breathe easier in case of sinusitis:

In half a cup of Apple Cider Vinegar, add 1 tablespoon of Honey, this mixture take 1 teaspoon 3 times a day, also place 1 drop in each nostril, this makes the mucus looser and easier.

b) To calm pain and inflammation of the paranasal sinuses: Half a freshly parboiled peeled potato is placed inside a gauze, and thus warm it is placed on the part of the paranasal sinuses and the forehead, with taps on the affected areas of the face.

c) To increase defenses and prevent sinusitis from attacking, prepare the following recipe:

Ingredients:

- 01 Carrot.
- 01 Beetroot.
- 01 Sweet chili.
- 01 glass of water

Preparation:

Peel the carrot and the beet, chop it into pieces, add it to the blender, along with the sweet chili, blend. Take on an empty stomach once a day, if possible take it all year round to keep the body's defenses high.

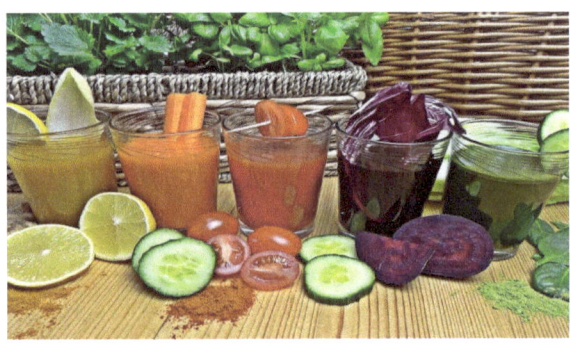

d) It is also recommended to take **Fenugreek in capsules**, (the content is yellow, this must be kept in mind when buying it to acquire the correct one), take one capsule daily, since it is a special herb that will help us assimilate the nutrients contained in the foods we are consuming and therefore the defenses of our organism increase.

e) Also prepare an infusion with Eucalyptus, Rosemary and Thyme, once it boils, we take it out of the fire, we lean with a towel around our head, in order to breathe the vapors that this infusion emanates, this will help us breathe better and decongest ourselves.

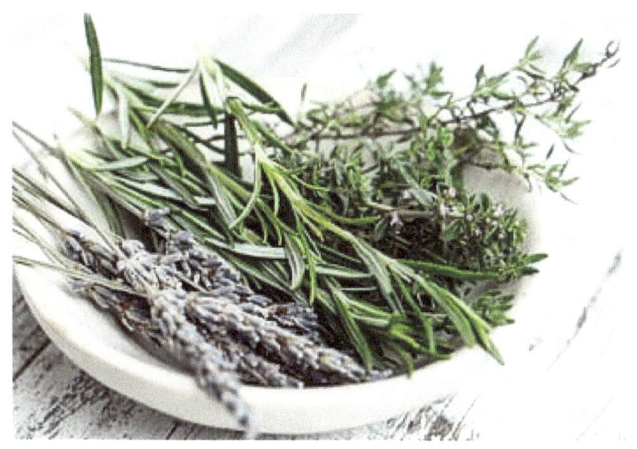

www.ingramcontent.com/pod-product-compliance
Lightning Source LLC
Chambersburg PA
CBHW041948240526
45473CB00036B/2784